Comfort Food Breakfast Guide for Beginners

50+ super simple comfort food recipes to start the day with

Johanna Reggie

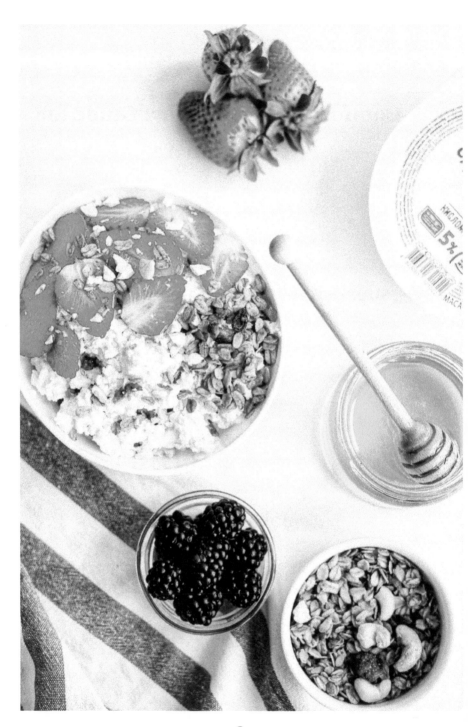

indirect, which are incurred as a result of the use of information contained within this document, including, but not limited to, — errors, omissions, or inaccuracies.

Table of Contents

Healthy Braised Kale

Preparation Time: 10 minutes | Cooking Time: 5 minutes | Servings: 6

Ingredients:

1 lb kale, chopped

1 tsp garlic, minced

1 onion, sliced

2 tbsp olive oil

14.5 oz can stew tomatoes

1 cup vegetable broth

1/4 tsp pepper

1 tsp salt

Directions:

Add oil into the inner pot of Pressure Pot duo crisp and set pot on sauté mode.

Add onion and sauté for 3-4 minutes.

Add remaining ingredients and stir well.

Seal the pot with a pressure-cooking lid and cook on high for 1 minute.

Once done, allow to release pressure naturally. Remove lid.

Stir and serve.

Nutrition:

Calories 110, Fat 5g, Carbohydrates 13g, Sugar 3g, Protein 4g, Cholesterol 0mg.

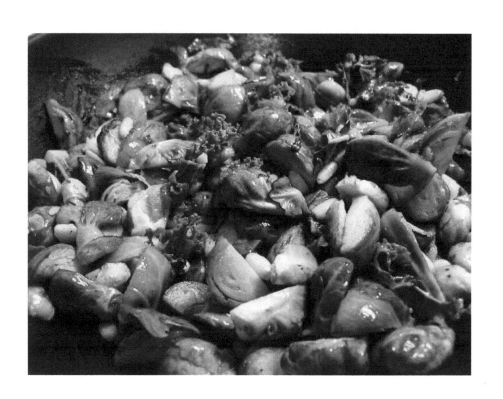

Sausage, Spinach & Broccoli Frittata

Preparation time: 15 minutes | Cooking Time: 30 minutes | Servings: 4

Ingredients:

1 teaspoon butter

6 turkey sausage links, cut into small pieces

1 cup broccoli florets, cut into small pieces

½ cup fresh spinach, chopped up

6 eggs

1/8 teaspoon hot sauce

2 tablespoons half-and-half

1/8 teaspoon garlic salt

Salt and ground black pepper, as required

¾ cup cheddar cheese, shredded

Directions:

In a skillet, melt the butter over medium heat and cook the sausage for about 7-8 minutes or until browned.

Add the broccoli and cook for about 3-4 minutes.

Add the spinach and cook for about 2-3 minutes.

Remove from the heat and set aside to cool slightly.

Meanwhile, in a bowl, add the eggs, half-and-half, hot sauce, garlic salt, salt, and black pepper, and beat until well combined.

Add the cheese and stir to combine.

In the bottom of a lightly greased pan, place the broccoli mixture and the egg mixture.

Press the "power button" of the air fry oven and turn the dial to select the "air bake" mode.

Press the time button and again turn the dial to set the cooking time to 15 minutes.

Now push the temp button and rotate the dial to set the temperature at 400° F.

Press the "start/pause" button to start.

When the unit beeps to show that it is preheated, open the lid.

Arrange pan over the "wire rack" and insert in the oven.

Cut into equal-sized wedges and serve hot.

Nutrition:

Calories 339, Total fat 27.4g, Saturated fat 11.6g, Cholesterol 229mg, Sodium 596mg, Total carbs 3.7g, Fiber 0.7g, Sugar 1.5g, Protein 19.6g.

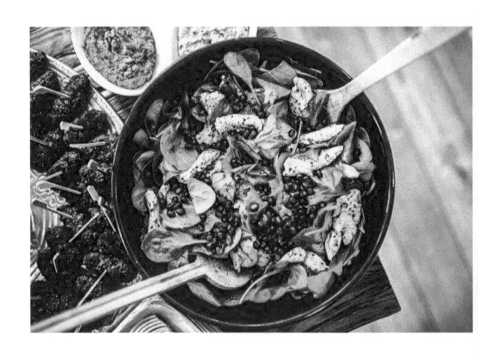

Sausage & Scallion Frittata

Preparation time: 15 minutes | Cooking Time: 20 minutes | Servings: 2

Ingredients:

¼ lb. Cooked breakfast sausage, crumbled

½ cup cheddar cheese, shredded

4 eggs, beaten lightly

2 scallions, chopped

Pinch of cayenne pepper

Directions:

In a bowl, add the sausage, cheese, eggs, scallion, and cayenne and mix until well combined.

Place the mixture into a greased baking pan.

Press the "power button" of the air fry oven and turn the dial to select the "air fry" mode.

Press the time button and again turn the dial to set the cooking time to 20 minutes.

Now push the temp button and rotate the dial to set the temperature at 360° F.

Press the "start/pause" button to start.

When the unit beeps to show that it is preheated, open the lid.

Arrange pan over the "wire rack" and insert in the oven.

Cut into equal-sized wedges and serve hot.

Nutrition:

Calories 437, Total fat 32.4g, Saturated fat 13.9g, Cholesterol 405mg, Sodium 726mg, Total carbs 2.2g, Fiber 0.4g, Sugar 1.2g, Protein 29.4g.

Trout Frittata

Preparation time: 15 minutes | Cooking Time: 25 minutes | Servings: 4

Ingredients:

1 tablespoon olive oil

1 onion, sliced

6 eggs

½ tablespoon horseradish sauce

2 tablespoons crème Fraiche

2 hot-smoked trout fillets, chopped

¼ cup fresh dill, chopped

Directions:

In a skillet, heat the oil over medium heat and cook the onion for about 4-5 minutes.

Remove from the heat and set aside.

Meanwhile, in a bowl, add the eggs, horseradish sauce, and crème Fraiche and mix well.

In the bottom of a baking pan, place the cooked onion and top with the egg mixture, followed by trout.

Press the "power button" of the air fry oven and turn the dial to select the "air fry" mode.

Press the time button and again turn the dial to set the cooking time to 20 minutes.

Now push the temp button and rotate the dial to set the temperature at 320° F.

Press the "start/pause" button to start.

When the unit beeps to show that it is preheated, open the lid.

Arrange pan over the "wire rack" and insert in the oven.

Cut into equal-sized wedges and serve with the garnishing of dill.

Nutrition:

Calories 258, Total fat 15.7g, Saturated fat 3.9g, Cholesterol 288mg, Sodium 141mg, Total carbs 5.1g, Fiber 1g, Sugar 1.8g, Protein 24.4g.

Mini Macaroni Quiches

Preparation time: 15 minutes | Cooking Time: 20 minutes | Servings: 4

Ingredients:

1 shortcrust pastry

½ cup leftover macaroni n' cheese

2 tablespoons plain Greek yogurt

1 teaspoon garlic puree

11 oz. Milk

2 large eggs

2 tablespoons parmesan cheese, grated

Directions:

Dust 4 ramekins with a little flour.

Line the bottom of prepared ramekins with shortcrust pastry.

In a bowl, mix macaroni, yogurt, and garlic.

Transfer the macaroni mixture between ramekins about ¾ full.

In a small bowl, add the milk and eggs and beat well.

Place the egg mixture over the macaroni mixture and top with the cheese evenly.

Press the "power button" of the air fry oven and turn the dial to select the "air fry" mode.

Press the time button and again turn the dial to set the cooking time to 20 minutes.

19

Now push the temp button and rotate the dial to set the temperature at 355° F.

Press the "start/pause" button to start.

When the unit beeps to show that it is preheated, open the lid.

Arrange the ramekins over the "wire rack" and insert them in the oven.

Serve hot.

Nutrition:

Calories 209, Total fat 10.4g, Saturated fat 2.9g, Cholesterol 102mg, Sodium 135mg, Total carbs 19.1g, Fiber 0.6g, Sugar 4.6g, Protein 9.6g.

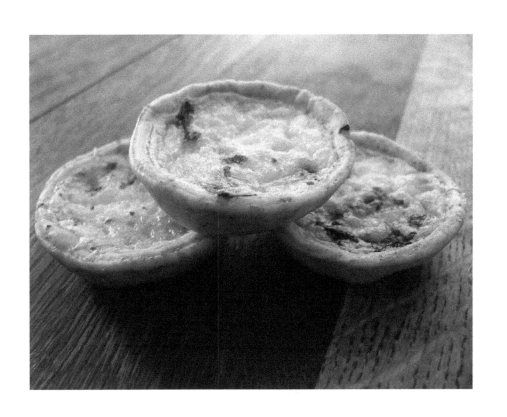

Tomato Quiche

Preparation time: 15 minutes | Cooking Time: 30 minutes | Servings: 2

Ingredients:

4 eggs

¼ cup onion, chopped

½ cup tomatoes, chopped

½ cup milk

1 cup gouda cheese, shredded

Salt, as required

Directions:

In a small baking pan, add all the ingredients and mix well.

Press the "power button" of the air fry oven and turn the dial to select the "air fry" mode.

Press the time button and again turn the dial to set the cooking time to 30 minutes.

Now push the temp button and rotate the dial to set the temperature at 340° F.

Press the "start/pause" button to start.

When the unit beeps to show that it is preheated, open the lid.

Arrange pan over the "wire rack" and insert in the oven.

Cut into equal-sized wedges and serve.

Nutrition:

Calories 247, Total fat 16.1g, Saturated fat 7.5g, Cholesterol 332mg, Sodium 417mg, Total carbs 7.3g, Fiber 0.9g, Sugar 5.2g, Protein 18.6g.

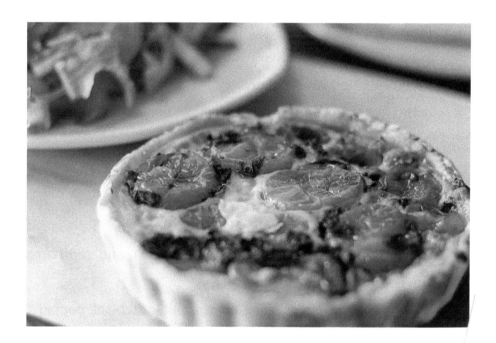

Chicken & Broccoli Quiche

Preparation time: 15 minutes | Cooking Time: 12 minutes | Servings: 2

Ingredients:

½ of frozen ready-made pie crust

¼ tablespoon olive oil

1 small egg

3 tablespoons cheddar cheese, grated

1½ tablespoons whipping cream

Salt and freshly ground black pepper, as needed

3 tablespoons boiled broccoli, chopped

2 tablespoons cooked chicken, chopped

Directions:

Cut 1 (5-inch round) from the pie crust.

Arrange the pie crust round in a small pie pan and gently, press in the bottom and sides.

In a bowl, mix the egg, cheese, cream, salt, and black pepper.

Pour the egg mixture over the dough base and top with the broccoli and chicken.

Press the "power button" of the air fry oven and turn the dial to select the "air fry" mode.

Press the time button and again turn the dial to set the cooking time to 12 minutes.

Now push the temp button and rotate the dial to set the temperature at 390° F.

Press the "start/pause" button to start.

When the unit beeps to show that it is preheated, open the lid.

Arrange pan over the "wire rack" and insert in the oven.

Cut into equal-sized wedges and serve.

Nutrition:

Calories 197, Total fat 15g, Saturated fat 5.9g, Cholesterol 99mg, Sodium 184mg, Total carbs 7.4g, Fiber 0.4g, Sugar 0.9g, Protein 8.6 g.

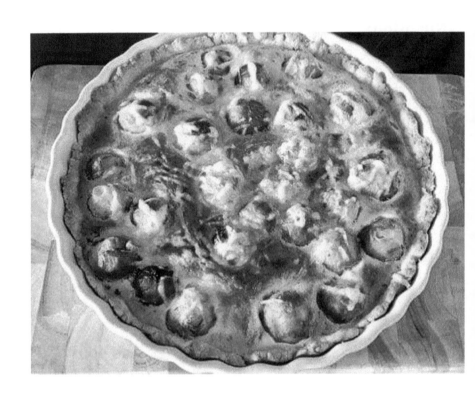

Eggplant and Spinach Frittata

Preparation time: 25 minutes | Cooking Time: 30 minutes | Servings: 4

Ingredients:

6 eggs; whisked

8 oz. Spinach; torn

1 eggplant; cubed

1 tbsp. Chives; chopped.

Cooking spray

Salt and black pepper to taste.

Directions:

Take a bowl and mix the eggs with the rest of the ingredients except the cooking spray and whisk well.

Grease a pan that fits your air fryer with the cooking spray, pour the frittata mix, spread and put the pan in the machine

Cook at 380°F for 20 minutes, divide between plates and serve for breakfast.

Nutrition:

Calories 240, Fat 8g, Fiber 3g, Carbs 6g, Protein 12g.

Zucchini and Artichokes Mix

Preparation time: 25 minutes | Cooking Time: 30 minutes | Servings: 4

Ingredients:

8 oz. Canned artichokes drained and chopped.

2 tomatoes; cut into quarters

4 eggs; whisked

4 spring onions; chopped.

2 zucchinis; sliced

Cooking spray

Salt and black pepper to taste.

Directions:

Grease a pan with cooking spray and mix all the other ingredients inside.

Put the pan in the air fryer and cook at 350°F for 20 minutes.

Divide between plates and serve

Nutrition:

Calories 210, Fat 11g, Fiber 3g, Carbs 4g, Protein 6g.

Tuna and Spring Onions Salad

Preparation time: 20 minutes | Cooking Time: 30 minutes | Servings: 4

Ingredients:

14 oz. Canned tuna, drained and flaked

2 spring onions; chopped.

1 cup arugula

1 tbsp. Olive oil

A pinch of salt and black pepper

Directions:

In a bowl, all the ingredients except the oil and the arugula and whisk.

Preheat the air fryer over 360°F, add the oil and grease it.

Pour the tuna mix, stir well and cook for 15 minutes

In a salad bowl, combine the arugula with the tuna mix, toss and serve.

Nutrition:

Calories 212, Fat 8g, Fiber 3g, Carbs 5g, Protein 8g.

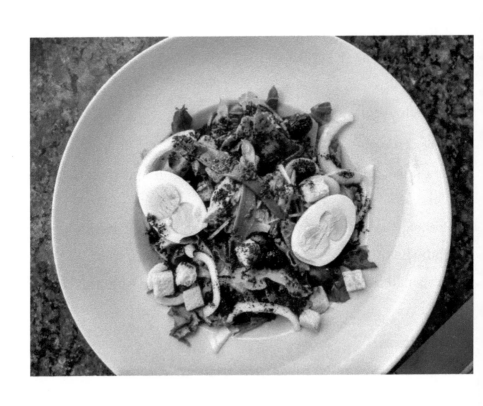

Cheesy Sausage Balls

Preparation time: 22 minutes | Cooking Time: 30 minutes | Servings: 16 balls

Ingredients:

1 lb. Pork breakfast sausage

1 large egg.

1 oz. Full-fat cream cheese; softened.

½ cup shredded cheddar cheese

Directions:

Mix all ingredients in a large bowl. Form into sixteen (1-inch balls).

Place the balls into the air fryer basket.

Adjust the temperature to 400° F and set the timer for 12 minutes.

Shake the basket two-or three-times during cooking

Sausage balls will be browned on the outside and have an internal temperature of at least 145° F when completely cooked.

Nutrition:

Calories 424, Protein 22.8g, Fiber 0.0g, Fat 32.2g, Carbs 1.6g.

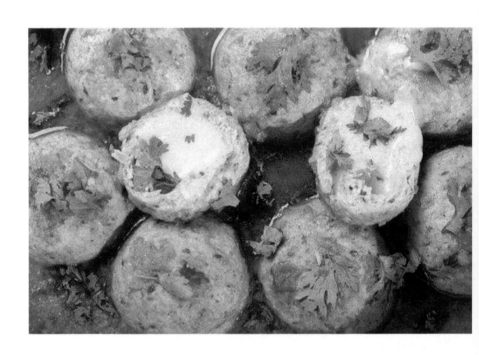

Cinnamon Banana Buckwheat Porridge

Preparation Time: 5 Minutes | Cooking Time: 5 Minutes | Servings: 2

Ingredients:

1/2 cup buckwheat groats, rinse

2 tbsp raisins

1/2 banana, sliced

1 1/2 cups almond milk

1/4 tsp vanilla

1/2 tsp cinnamon

Directions:

Add all ingredients into the Pressure Pot and stir well to combine.

Seal pot with lid and cook on high pressure for 5 minutes.

Allow releasing pressure naturally then open the lid.

Stir and serve.

Nutrition:

Calories 571, Carbohydrates 45.6g, Protein 8.5g, Fat 44g, Sugar 15.8g, Sodium 32mg.

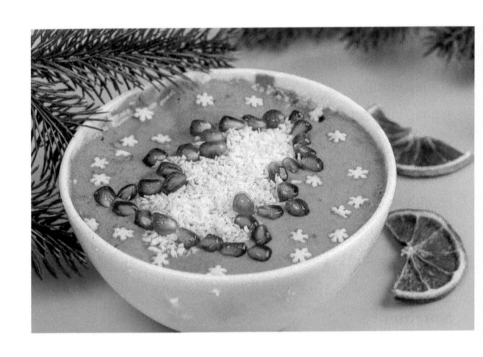

Spinach and Mushroom Frittata

Preparation Time: 10Minutes | Cooking Time:7Minutes | Servings: 4

Ingredients:

1 cup fresh baby spinach

8 large eggs

6 bacon slices, diced

Pinch of salt, pepper

1 cup of water

Directions:

Press "Sauté" on Pressure Pot. Add diced bacon. Cook until brown. Set aside. Turn off the "Sauté" function.

In a large bowl, add eggs, spinach, bacon, salt, pepper. Stir until combined.

Grease 4 individual ramekins with nonstick cooking spray. Divide egg mixture evenly between ramekins. Cover with aluminum foil.

Add 1 cup water and trivet to Pressure Pot. Place ramekins on top.

Lock, seal lid. Press the "Manual" button. Cook on HIGH 5 minutes.

When done, naturally release pressure for 10 minutes, remove the lid. Serve.

Nutrition:

Calories 293, Fat 20.9g, Carbohydrates 3.2g, Dietary Fiber:1.3g, Protein 23.3g.

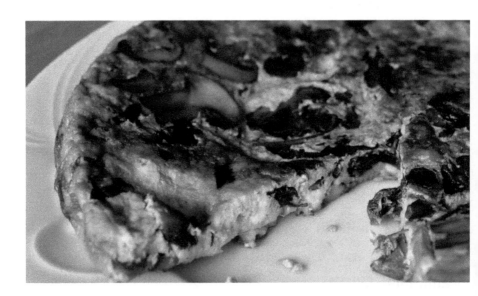

Mini Frittata

Preparation Time: 10 minutes | Cooking Time: 15 minutes | Servings: 4

Ingredients:

6 eggs

1/2 small onion, chopped

1/2 bell pepper, chopped

3 bacon slices, chopped

1/4 cup cheddar cheese, shredded

1/4 cup coconut milk

1/4 tsp black pepper

1/2 tsp sea salt

Directions:

Add bacon slices to the bottom of each silicone muffin mold.

Add chopped vegetables on top of the bacon.

In a bowl, whisk eggs with pepper and salt.

Pour egg mixture over vegetables.

Sprinkle shredded cheddar cheese on top.

Place silicone muffin molds into the Pressure Pot air fryer basket and place the basket in the pot.

Seal the pot with a pressure-cooking lid and select bake mode and cook at 350° F for 10-15 minutes.

Serve and enjoy.

Nutrition:

Calories 243, Fat 18.5g, Carbohydrates 3.7g, Sugar 2.2g, Protein 15.9g, Cholesterol 269mg.

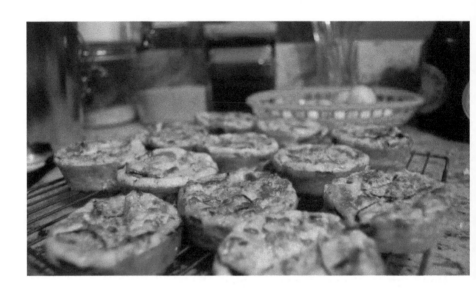

Spinach Frittata

Preparation Time: 10 minutes | Cooking Time: 15 minutes | Servings: 4

Ingredients:

6 eggs

1/4 cup bacon, cooked and chopped

1 tomato, chopped

1/4 tsp garlic powder

3/4 cup fresh spinach

1 tsp Italian seasoning

1 tbsp heavy cream

1/4 tsp pepper

1/4 tsp salt

Directions:

In a bowl, whisk eggs with spices and heavy cream.

Spray a 7-inch baking dish with cooking spray.

Add bacon, tomato, and spinach to the prepared dish.

Pour egg mixture over the bacon mixture. Cover dish with foil.

Pour 1 1/2 cups of water into the inner pot of the Pressure Pot then place steamer rack in the pot.

Place baking dish on top of the steamer rack.

Seal the pot with a pressure-cooking lid and cook on high for 15 minutes.

Once done, release pressure using a quick release. Remove lid.

Serve and enjoy.

Nutrition:

Calories 122, Fat 8.9g, Carbohydrates 1.8g, Sugar 1.1g, Protein 9.2g, Cholesterol 253mg.

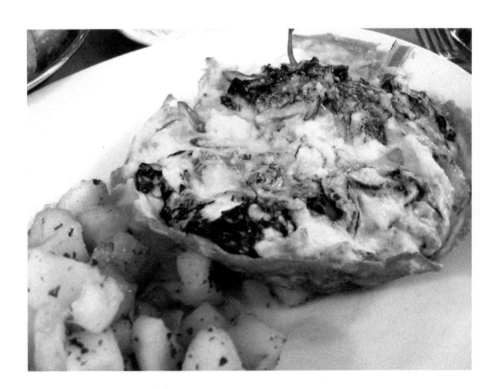

Mushroom Frittata

Preparation Time: 10 minutes | Cooking Time: 15 minutes | Servings: 2

Ingredients:

4 eggs

1 1/2 cups water

1/4 tsp garlic powder

4 oz mushrooms, sliced

1/8 tsp white pepper

1/8 tsp onion powder

2 tsp heavy cream

2 Swiss cheese slices, cut each slice into 4 pieces

1/4 tsp salt

Directions:

In a bowl, whisk eggs with spices and heavy cream.

Spray a 7-inch baking dish with cooking spray.

Add sliced mushrooms to the dish then pour egg mixture over the mushrooms.

Arrange cheese slices on top of the mushroom and egg mixture.

Cover dish with foil.

Pour 1 1/2 cups of water into the Pressure Pot then place steamer rack in the pot.

Place dish on top of the steamer rack.

Seal the pot with a pressure-cooking lid and cook on high for 15 minutes.

Once done, release pressure using a quick release. Remove lid. Serve and enjoy.

Nutrition:

Calories 264, Fat 18.5g, Carbohydrates 4.6g, Sugar 2.2g, Protein 20.6g, Cholesterol 360mg.

Tomato Mozzarella Quiche

Preparation Time: 10 minutes | Cooking Time: 30 minutes | Servings: 6

Ingredients:

8 eggs

1 red pepper, chopped

1/2 cup almond flour

1/2 cup almond milk

1 1/2 cup mozzarella cheese, shredded

2 tbsp green onions, chopped

1 cup tomatoes, chopped

1/4 tsp pepper

1/4 tsp salt

Directions:

Pour 1 1/2 cups of water into the Pressure Pot then place steamer rack in the pot.

In a large bowl, whisk eggs, almond flour, milk, pepper, and salt. Add vegetables and cheese and stir to combine.

Pour egg mixture into the baking dish. Cover the dish with foil and place it on top of the steamer rack.

Seal the pot with a pressure-cooking lid and cook on high for 30 minutes.

Once done, allow to release pressure naturally for 10 minutes then release remaining pressure using a quick release. Remove lid.

Serve and enjoy.

Nutrition:

Calories 219, Fat 16.4g, Carbohydrates 6.7g, Sugar 3g, Protein 12.4g, Cholesterol 222mg.

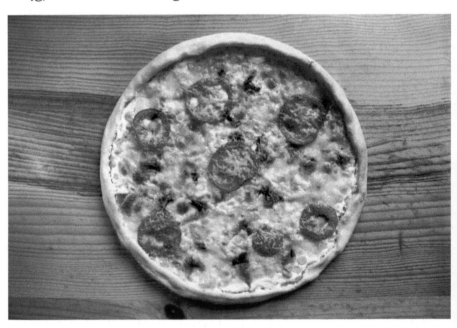

Lemon Butter Brussels sprouts

Preparation Time: 10 minutes | Cooking Time: 5 minutes | Servings: 4

Ingredients:

1 lb Brussels sprouts, trimmed and washed

1 fresh lemon juice

1/4 cup parmesan cheese, grated

1/4 tsp garlic powder

2 tbsp butter

1 cup of water

Directions:

Pour water into the inner pot of Pressure Pot duo crisp.

Add Brussels sprouts into the steamer basket and place the basket in the pot.

Seal the pot with a pressure-cooking lid and cook on high for 2 minutes.

Once done, release pressure using a quick release. Remove lid.

Drain Brussels sprouts well and place in a mixing bowl.

Clean the pot. Add butter into the pot and set the pot on sauté mode.

Add cooked Brussels sprouts, garlic powder, and lemon juice and sauté for 2-3 minutes.

Top with cheese and serve.

Nutrition:

Calories 123, Fat 7.6g, Carbohydrates 10.9g, Sugar 2.7g, Protein 6.1g, Cholesterol 20mg.

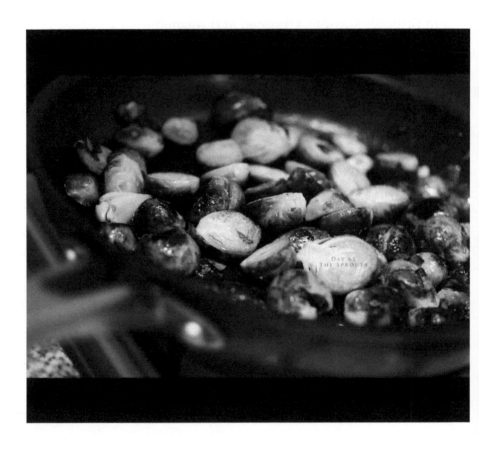

Easy Omelet

Preparation time: 10 minutes | Cooking Time: 30 minutes | Servings: 4

Ingredients:

6 eggs, whisked

A pinch of black pepper

½ cup coconut cream

6 ounces low-sodium bacon, chopped

½ cup red bell peppers, chopped

4 spring onions, chopped

¾ cup low-fat cheese, shredded

1 and ½ cups of water

Cooking spray

Directions:

In a bowl, mix the eggs with black pepper, cream, bacon, bell peppers, onions, and cheese and whisk well.

Grease a pan that fits your Pressure Pot with cooking spray and pour the omelet mix inside.

Add the water to your Pressure Pot, add steamer basket, add the pan with the omelet mix, cover and cook on High for 30 minutes.

Slice the omelet, divide it between plates, and serve for breakfast.

Enjoy!

Nutrition:

Calories 231, fat 4g, fiber 5g, carbs 16g, Protein 6g.

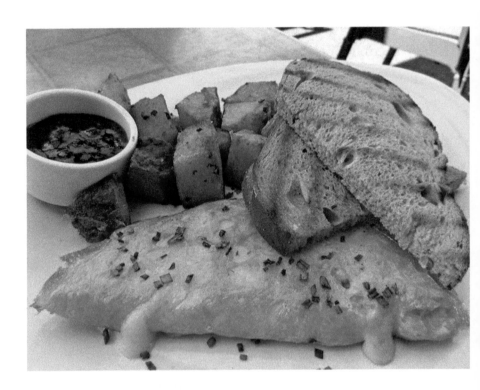

Hard-Boiled Eggs

Preparation time: 20 minutes | Cooking Time: 30 minutes | Servings: 4

Ingredients:

1 cup of water

4 large eggs.

Directions:

Place eggs into a 4-cup round baking-safe dish and pour water over eggs.

Place dish into the air fryer basket.

Adjust the temperature to 300° F and set the timer for 18 minutes.

Store cooked eggs in the refrigerator until ready to use or peel and eat warm.

Nutrition:

Calories 77, Protein 6.3g, Fiber 0.0g, Fat 4.4g, Carbs 0.6g.

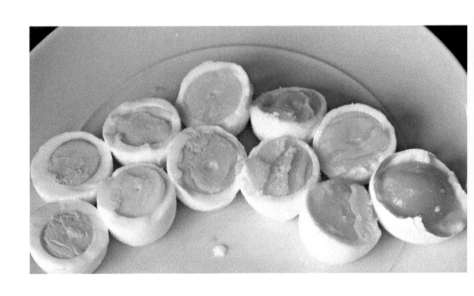

Stuffed Poblanos

Preparation time: 30 minutes | Cooking Time: 30 minutes | Servings: 4

Ingredients:

½ lb. Spicy ground pork breakfast sausage

4 large poblano peppers

4 large eggs.

½ cup full-fat sour cream.

4 oz. Full-fat cream cheese; softened.

¼ cup canned diced tomatoes and green chiles, drained

8 tbsp. Shredded pepper jack cheese

Directions:

In a medium skillet over medium heat, crumble and brown the ground sausage until no pink remains. Remove sausage and drain the fat from the pan.

Crack eggs into the pan, scramble, and cook until no longer runny

Place cooked sausage in a large bowl and fold in cream cheese.

Mix in diced tomatoes and chiles. Gently fold in eggs

Cut a 4"–5" slit in the top of each poblano, removing the seeds and white membrane with a small knife.

Separate the filling into four serving and spoon carefully into each pepper.

Top each with 2 tbsp. Pepper jack cheese

Place each pepper into the air fryer basket.

Adjust the temperature to 350° F and set the timer for 15 minutes.

Peppers will be soft and cheese will be browned when ready.

Serve immediately with sour cream on top.

Nutrition:

Calories 489, Protein 22.8g, Fiber 3.8g, Fat 35.6g, Carbs 12.6g.

Yogurt Omelet

Preparation time: 25 minutes | Cooking Time: 30 minutes | Servings: 4

Ingredients:

1 ½ cups Greek yogurt

4 eggs; whisked

1 tbsp. Cilantro; chopped.

1 tbsp. Chives; chopped.

Cooking spray

Salt and black pepper to taste.

Directions:

Take a bowl and mix all the ingredients except the cooking spray and whisk well.

Now, take a pan that fits in your air fryer and grease it with the cooking spray, pour the eggs mix, spread well, put the pan into the machine, and cook the omelet at 360°F for 20 minutes.

Divide between plates and serve for breakfast

Nutrition:

Calories 221, Fat 14g, Fiber 4g, Carbs 6g, Protein 11g.

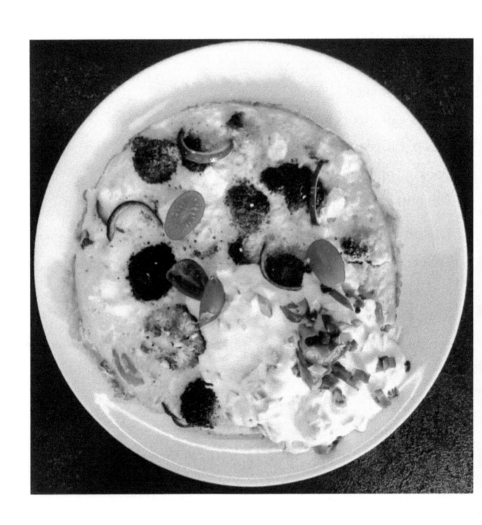

54

Pressure Pot Scrambled Eggs

Preparation Time: 2 minutes | Cooking Time: 3 minutes | Servings: 2

Ingredients:

2 eggs

1 tablespoon milk

Salt and pepper to taste

½ tablespoon butter

Directions:

Place a trivet or steamer basket inside the Pressure Pot and pour water over.

In a mixing bowl, combine the eggs and milk. Season with salt and pepper to taste.

Place the egg mixture into a heatproof bowl that will fit in the Pressure Pot.

Place the bowl with the egg mixture on the steamer basket.

Close the lid.

Press the Manual button and adjust the cooking time to 3 minutes.

Do natural pressure release. Once the lid is open, add the butter and use a fork to fluff the eggs until they look like they are scrambled.

Nutrition:

Calories 169, Carbohydrates 3.5g, Protein 9.7g, Fat 12.8g, Fiber 0.3g.

Pressure Pot Egg Custard

Preparation Time: 5 minutes | Cooking Time: 10 minutes | Servings: 2

Ingredients:

4 cups of milk

6 large eggs, beaten

¾ cup white sugar

1 teaspoon vanilla extract

A pinch of salt

¼ teaspoon ground cinnamon

Directions:

Place a trivet or steamer basket inside the Pressure Pot and pour water over.

In a mixing bowl, combine all ingredients. Whisk until well-combined.

Place the egg mixture into a baking dish that will fit inside the Pressure Pot. Cover with aluminum foil.

Place the baking dish with the egg mixture on the steamer basket.

Close the lid.

Press the Manual button and adjust the cooking time to 10 minutes.

Do natural pressure release.

Nutrition:

Calories 212, Carbohydrates 11.7g, Protein 8.6g, Fat 14.6g, Fiber 0.7g.

Green Beans and Olives

Preparation time: 25 minutes | Cooking Time: 15 minutes | Servings: 2

Ingredients:

1 cup green beans; halved

4 eggs; whisked

2 spring onions; chopped.

¼ tsp. Cumin, ground

Salt and black pepper to taste.

Directions:

Preheat the air fryer at 360°F, add all the ingredients, toss, cover, cook for 20 minutes,

Divide between plates and serve for breakfast

Nutrition:

Calories 183, Fat 8g, Fiber 2g, Carbs 3g, Protein 7g.

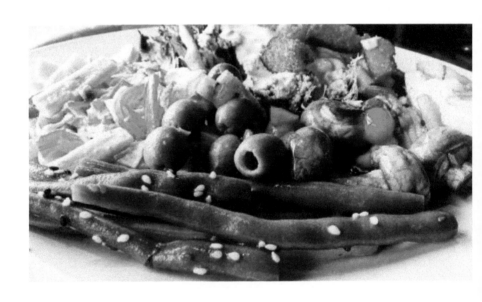

Zucchini and Watercress Salad

Preparation time: 19 minutes | Cooking Time: 15 minutes | Servings: 2

Ingredients:

2 cups zucchini, roughly cubed

1 cup parmesan cheese; grated

1 cup watercress; torn

1 tbsp. Olive oil

Cooking spray

Directions:

Now, take a pan that fits in your air fryer and grease it with the cooking spray, add all the ingredients except the cheese, sprinkle the cheese on top and cook at 390°F for 15 minutes

Divide into bowls and serve for breakfast.

Nutrition:

Calories 202, Fat 11g, Fiber 3g, Carbs 5g, Protein 4g.

Tomatoes and Olives Eggs

Preparation time: 20 minutes | Cooking Time: 15 minutes | Servings: 4

Ingredients:

1 cup kalamata olives, pitted and sliced

4 eggs; whisked

1 cup cherry tomatoes; cubed

A pinch of salt and black pepper

Cooking spray

Directions:

Grease the air fryer with cooking spray, add all the ingredients, toss, cover, and cook at 365°F for 10 minutes.

Divide between plates and serve for breakfast

Nutrition:

Calories 182, Fat 6g, Fiber 2g, Carbs 4g, Protein 8g.

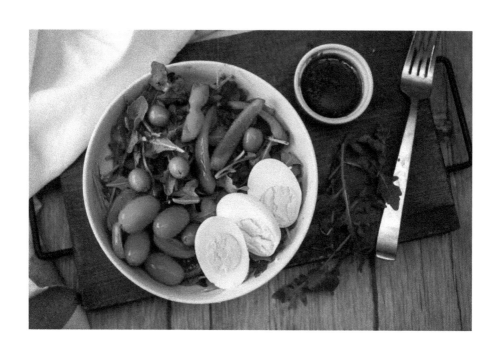

Mix Veggie Egg Cups

Preparation Time: 10 minutes | Cooking Time: 14 minutes | Servings: 4

Ingredients:

4 eggs

1 cup cheddar cheese, shredded

1 cup mixed vegetables, diced

1 tbsp cilantro, chopped

4 tbsp half and half

Pepper

Salt

Directions:

In a mixing bowl, whisk eggs with cilantro, half and half, vegetables, 1/2 cup cheese, pepper, and salt.

Pour egg mixture into the four ramekins.

Place the dehydrating tray in a multi-level air fryer basket and place basket in the Pressure Pot.

Place ramekins on dehydrating tray.

Seal pot with air fryer lid and select air fry mode then set the temperature to 320° F and timer for 12 minutes.

Top with remaining 1/2 cup cheese and air fry for 2 minutes more.

Serve and enjoy.

Nutrition:

Calories 211, Fat 15.5g, Carbohydrates 4.1g, Sugar 1.3g, Protein 13.8g, Cholesterol 199mg.

Egg Soufflé

Preparation Time: 5 minutes | Cooking Time: 8 minutes | Servings: 2

Ingredients:

2 eggs

2 tbsp heavy cream

1 tbsp parsley, chopped

1/4 tsp pepper

Salt

Directions:

In a bowl, whisk eggs with remaining gradients.

Spray two ramekins with cooking spray.

Place the dehydrating tray in a multi-level air fryer basket and place basket in the Pressure Pot.

Pour egg mixture into the prepared ramekins and place them on a dehydrating tray.

Seal pot with air fryer lid and select air fry mode then set the temperature to 390° F and timer for 8 minutes.

Serve and enjoy.

Nutrition:

Calories 116, Fat 10g, Carbohydrates 1.1g, Sugar 0.4g, Protein 5.9g, Cholesterol 184mg.

Veggie Egg Soufflé

Preparation Time: 10 minutes | Cooking Time: 20 minutes | Servings: 4

Ingredients:

4 large eggs

1/2 cup broccoli florets, chopped

1/2 cup mushrooms, chopped

1 tsp onion powder

1 tsp garlic powder

Directions:

Spray four ramekins with cooking spray and set them aside.

In a bowl, whisk eggs with onion powder, and garlic powder.

Add mushrooms and broccoli and stir well.

Place the dehydrating tray in a multi-level air fryer basket and place basket in the Pressure Pot.

Pour egg mixture into the prepared ramekins and place them on a dehydrating tray.

Seal pot with air fryer lid and select air fry mode then set the temperature to 350° F and timer for 20 minutes.

Serve and enjoy.

Nutrition:

Calories 82, Fat 5.1g, Carbohydrates 2.4g, Sugar 1.1g, Protein 7.1g, Cholesterol 186mg.

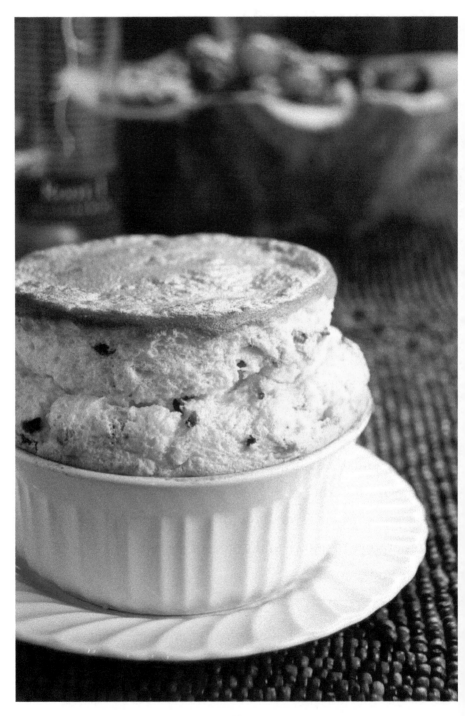

Spicy Bok Choy And Tomatoes Soup Bowls

Preparation Time: 30 minutes, | Cooking Time: 20 minutes | Servings: 4

Ingredients:

1 ½ cups Veggie stock

cups have Roughly torn Bok Choy

Tomatoes: cubed

1 tbsp sweet paprika

1 tbsp Coconut aminos

A pinch of salt and black pepper

tbsp Grated ginger

Minced garlic cloves

Directions:

Combine all the ingredients in the Pressure Pot and seal the lid to cook for 20 minutes at high pressure.

Natural release the pressure for 10 minutes, share into bowls, and serve.

Nutrition:

Calories 89, Fat 6.8g, Carbs 6.1g, Protein 1.7g, Fiber 2.1g.

Avocado Tussle with White Mushrooms

Preparation Time: 30 minutes, | Cooking Time: 20 minutes | Servings: 4

Ingredients:

1 cup baby arugula

½ cup Veggie stock

Avocados; pitted and cubed

½ Ib. Sliced white mushrooms

1 tbsp Chopped chives

A pinch of salt and black pepper

1 tbsp Balsamic vinegar

1 tbsp Olive oil

Directions:

Press 'Sauté' on the Pressure Pot and pour in the oil. When hot, add the mushrooms to cook for 4 minutes.

Gently pour in the veggie stock, vinegar, salt and pepper, and chives. Stir and seal the lid to cook for 15 minutes at high pressure.

Natural release the pressure for 10 minutes. Pour it inside a salad bowl and mix in the baby arugula and the avocado. Serve.

Nutrition:

Calories 250, Fat 23.3g, Carbs 7.6g, Protein 3.8g, Fiber 6.4g.

Creamy Salmon with Eggs and Cilantro

Preparation Time: 22 minutes, | Cooking Time: 20 minutes | Servings: 4

Ingredients:

oz Smoked salmon; skinless and boneless: cut into strips

Eggs

1 tbsp Chopped cilantro

1 tbsp Chopped chives

½ cup Coconut cream

A pinch of salt and black pepper

Cooking spray

Directions:

Whisk the salmon, cilantro, eggs, chives, cream, salt, and pepper in a bowl.

Coat the Pressure Pot with the cooking spray and pour the creamy egg mixture into the pot. Seal the lid to cook for 12 minutes on high pressure.

Natural release the pressure for 10 minutes, share, and serve.

Nutrition:

Calories 167, fat 12.9g, carbs 2.1g, Protein 11.4g, fiber 0.7g.

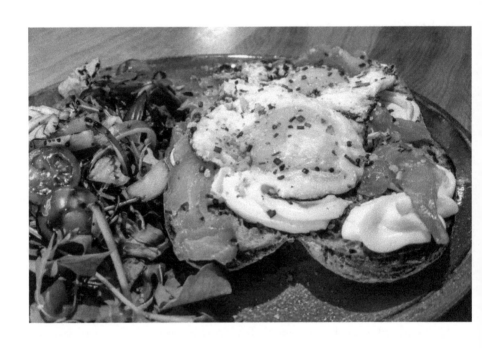

Herbed Mushroom

Preparation Time: 30 minutes, | Cooking Time: 20 minutes | Servings: 4

Ingredients:

1 Red bell pepper; cut into strips

1 ½ lb. Chopped brown mushrooms

tbsp Chicken stock

A pinch of salt and black pepper

1 tbsp Olive oil

½ tsp Garlic powder

½ tsp Dried basil

1 tsp Chopped rosemary

Directions:

Press 'Sauté' on the Pressure Pot and pour in the oil. When it is hot, add the mushrooms and cook for 5 minutes.

Mix in the red bell pepper, rosemary, chicken stock, dried basil, garlic powder, salt, and pepper then seal the lid to cook for 15 minutes at high pressure.

Natural release the pressure for 10 minutes, share into plates, and serve.

Nutrition:

Calories 42, fat 3.7g, carbs 2.7g, protein 0.4g, fiber 0.6g.

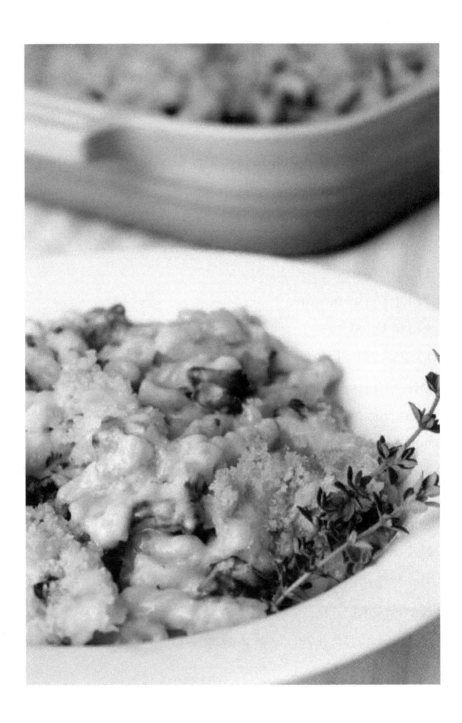

74

Creamy Walnuts and Cardamom Mousse

Preparation Time: 15 minutes. | Cooking Time: 20 minutes | Servings: 2

Ingredients:

1 tsp ground cardamom

½ cup Chopped walnuts

1 tsp Swerve

tbsp Almond meal

1 ½ cups Coconut cream

Directions:

Combine the cardamom, almond meal, walnuts, cream, and swerve in the Pressure Pot and seal the lid to cook for 10 minutes at high pressure.

Quick-release the pressure for 5 minutes, share into bowls, and serve.

Nutrition:

Calories 231, fat 21.9g, carbs 5.1g, protein 8.9g, fiber 3.2g.

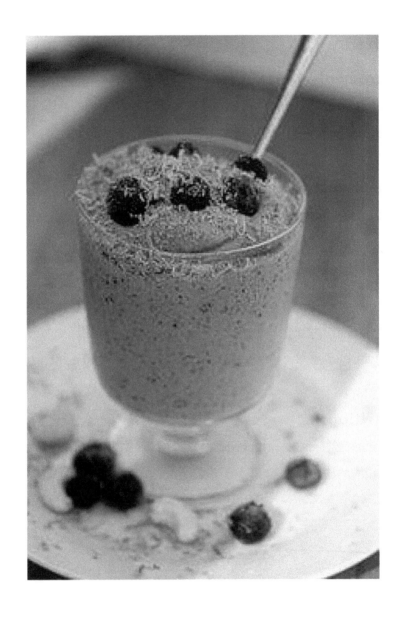

Cheesy Chili Eggs

Preparation Time: 20 minutes | Cooking Time: 20 minutes | Servings: 4

Ingredients:

1 cup shredded cheddar cheese

Whisked eggs

2 tbsp Chopped basil

A pinch of salt and black pepper

Cooking spray

1 tsp Chili powder

Directions:

Coat the Pressure Pot with the cooking spray and mix in the basil, chili powder, cheddar cheese, eggs, salt, and pepper then seal the lid to cook for 15 minutes at high pressure.

Quick-release the pressure for 5 minutes, share into plates, and serve.

Nutrition:

Calories 180, fat 14g, carbs 1.1g, protein 12.7g, fiber 0.3g.

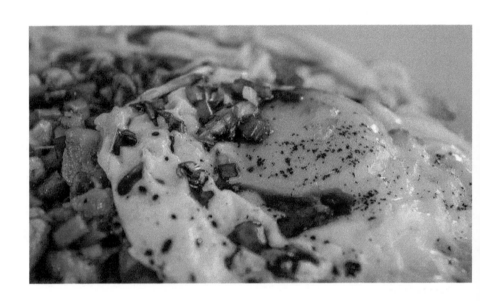

Nutty Blueberries Mix

Preparation Time: 13 minutes, | Cooking Time: 20 minutes | Servings: 6

Ingredients:

½ cup Chopped walnuts

½ cup Chopped almonds

1 cup Blueberries

2 tsp Swerve

1 cup Coconut cream

1 tsp Vanilla extract

Directions:

Mix all the ingredients in the Pressure Pot and seal the lid to cook for 8 minutes on high pressure.

Quick-release the pressure for 5 minutes, share into bowls, and serve.

Nutrition:

Calories 218, fat 19.7g, carbs 5.8g, protein 5.3g, fiber 3.2g.

Tomato Egg Muffins

Preparation Time: 10 minutes | Cooking Time: 20 minutes | Servings: 6

Ingredients:

2 eggs

4 egg whites

1/4 cup cheddar cheese, shredded

1 tbsp fresh parsley, chopped

1/4 cup olives, diced

1/4 cup onion, diced

1/4 cup tomatoes, diced

1/2 cup almond milk

Pepper

Salt

Directions:

In a mixing bowl, whisk eggs, egg whites, milk, pepper, and salt.

Add cheese, parsley, olives, onion, and tomatoes and stir well.

Pour egg mixture into the 6 silicone muffin molds.

Place the dehydrating tray in a multi-level air fryer basket and place basket in the Pressure Pot.

Place muffin molds on a dehydrating tray.

Seal pot with air fryer lid and select bake mode then set the temperature to 350° F and timer for 20 minutes.

Serve and enjoy.

Nutrition:

Calories 107, Fat 8.5g, Carbohydrates 2.6g, Sugar 1.4g, Protein 6.1g, Cholesterol 60mg.

Mac & Cheese

Preparation Time: 10 minutes | Cooking Time: 15 minutes | Servings: 4

Ingredients:

1 1/2 cups elbow macaroni, cooked and drained

1/4 tsp garlic powder

8 oz cheddar cheese, shredded

1/4 cup heavy cream

Pepper

Salt

Directions:

Spray baking dish with cooking spray.

Add macaroni, garlic powder, dry mustard, cheese, heavy cream, water, pepper, and salt to the prepared baking dish and stir well.

Place steam rack into the Pressure Pot then places baking dish on top of the rack.

Seal pot with air fryer lid and select air fry mode then set the temperature to 360° F and timer for 10-15 minutes.

Serve and enjoy.

Nutrition:

Calories 372, Fat 22.1g, Carbohydrates 24.6g, Sugar 1.2g, Protein 18.4g, Cholesterol 70mg.

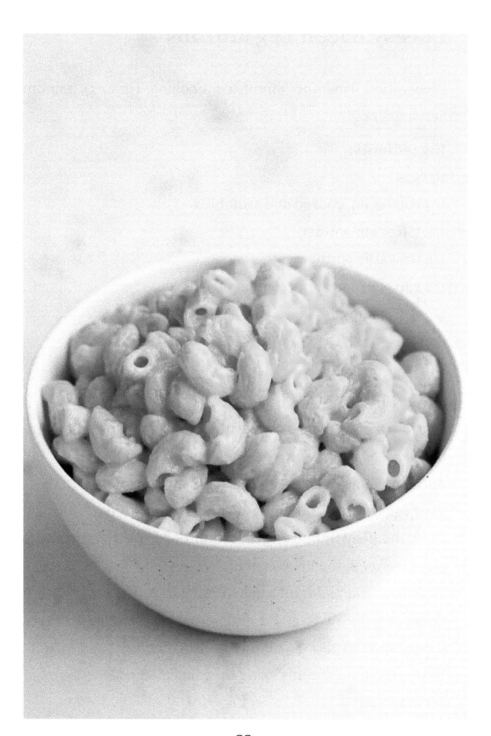

Cheesy Bacon Egg Muffins

Preparation Time: 10 minutes | Cooking Time: 15 minutes | Servings: 12

Ingredients:

10 eggs

1/3 cup bacon, cooked and crumbled

1/2 tsp onion powder

1/2 tsp garlic powder

1/2 cup cheddar cheese, shredded

1/3 cup cream cheese

Pepper

Salt

Directions:

In a large bowl, whisk eggs with onion powder, garlic powder, pepper, and salt.

Add remaining ingredients and stir everything well.

Pour egg mixture into the 12 silicone muffin molds.

Place the dehydrating tray in a multi-level air fryer basket and place basket in the Pressure Pot.

Place 6 muffin molds on a dehydrating tray.

Seal pot with air fryer lid and select bake mode then set the temperature to 380° F and timer for 15 minutes.

Bake remaining muffins using the same method.

Serve and enjoy.

Nutrition:

Calories 114, Fat 8.9g, Carbohydrates 0.7g, Sugar 0.4g, Protein 7.6g, Cholesterol 152mg.

Zucchini Muffins

Preparation Time: 10 minutes | Cooking Time: 25 minutes | Servings: 12

Ingredients:

1 egg

1/2 cup cheddar cheese, shredded

1/4 cup onion, diced

2 cups zucchini, shredded

Pepper

Salt

Directions:

In a bowl, whisk the egg with pepper and salt.

Add zucchini, cheese, and onion and stir everything well.

Pour egg mixture into the 12 silicone muffin molds.

Place the dehydrating tray in a multi-level air fryer basket and place basket in the Pressure Pot.

Place 6 muffin molds on a dehydrating tray.

Seal pot with air fryer lid and select bake mode then set the temperature to 350° F and timer for 25 minutes.

Bake remaining muffins using the same method.

Serve and enjoy.

Nutrition:

Calories 28, Fat 2g, Carbohydrates 1g, Sugar 0.5g, Protein 1.9g, Cholesterol 19mg.

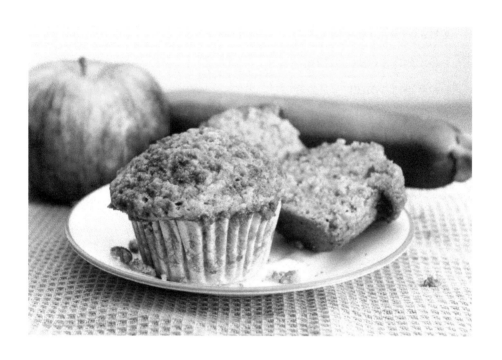

Chia Oatmeal

Preparation time: 10 minutes | Cooking Time: 15 minutes | Servings: 6

Ingredients:

1 cup steel-cut oatmeal

1/2 tsp vanilla

2 tbsp chia seeds

1 1/2 cups coconut milk

1 1/2 cup water

1/4 tsp sea salt

Directions:

Spray Pressure Pot from inside with cooking spray.

Add all ingredients into the Pressure Pot and stir well.

Seal pot with lid and cook on porridge mode for 15 minutes.

Once done then allow to release pressure naturally for 10 minutes then release using the quick-release method. Open the lid.

Stir well and serve.

Nutrition:

Calories 210, Fat 17.7g, Carbohydrates 11.8g, Sugar 2g, Protein 3.8g, Cholesterol 0mg.

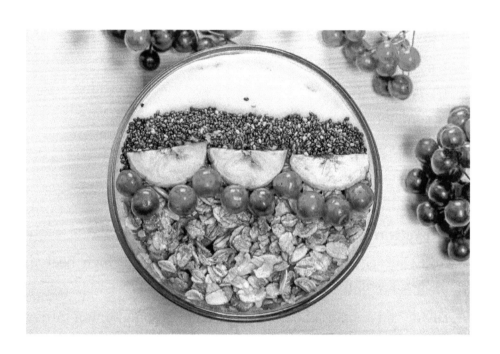

Sausage Breakfast Muffins

Preparation Time: 10 minutes | Cooking Time: 25 minutes | Servings: 6

Ingredients:

3 eggs

1/2 lb ground pork sausage

2 tbsp onion, minced

1/4 red pepper, diced

1/2 cup egg whites

1/4 cup mozzarella cheese

1/2 cup cheddar cheese

Pepper

Salt

Directions:

Add sausage to a pan and cook over medium-high heat until meat is no pink.

Divide red pepper, cheese, cooked sausages, and onion into each silicone muffin molds.

In a large bowl, whisk together egg whites, egg, pepper, and salt. Pour egg mixture into each muffin mold.

Place silicone muffin molds into the Pressure Pot air fryer basket and place the basket in the pot.

Seal the pot with an air fryer lid and select bake mode and cook at 350° F for 20-25 minutes.

Serve and enjoy.

Nutrition:

Calories 188, Fat 12g, Carbohydrates 2g, Sugar 0.7g, Protein 12g, Cholesterol 115 mg

Blueberry Lemon Oatmeal

Preparation time: 10 minutes | Cooking Time: 10 minutes | Servings: 6

Ingredients:

1 cup steel-cut oats

1/4 cup chia seeds

1 cup blueberries

1/2 tbsp lemon zest

2 tbsp sugar

1/2 cup half and half

3 cups of water

1 tbsp butter

Salt

Directions:

Add butter into the Pressure Pot and set the pot on sauté mode.

Add oats into the pot and stir well.

Add remaining ingredients and stir everything well.

Seal pot with lid and cook on manual high pressure for 10 minutes.

Once done then allow to release pressure naturally then open the lid.

Stir well and serve.

Nutrition:

Calories 130, Fat 5.6g, Carbohydrates 18.2g, Sugar 6.6g, Protein 2.8g, Cholesterol 13mg.

Breakfast Cobbler

Preparation time: 10 minutes | Cooking Time: 15 minutes | Servings: 2

Ingredients:

2 tbsp sunflower seeds

1/4 cup pecan

1/4 cup shredded coconut

1/2 tsp cinnamon

2 1/2 tbsp coconut oil

2 tbsp honey

1 plum, diced

1 apple, diced

1 pear, diced

Directions:

Add fruits, cinnamon, coconut oil, and honey into the Pressure Pot and stir well.

Seal pot with a lid and select steam mode and set timer for 10 minutes.

Once done then release pressure using the quick-release method then open the lid.

Transfer fruit mixture into the serving bowl.

Add sunflower seeds, pecans, and coconut into the pot and cook on sauté mode for 5 minutes.

Pour sunflower seed, pecans, and coconut mixture on top of fruit mixture.

Serve and enjoy.

Nutrition:

Calories 426, Fat 27.2g, Carbohydrates 50.9g, Sugar 40.1g, Protein 2.6g, Cholesterol 0mg.

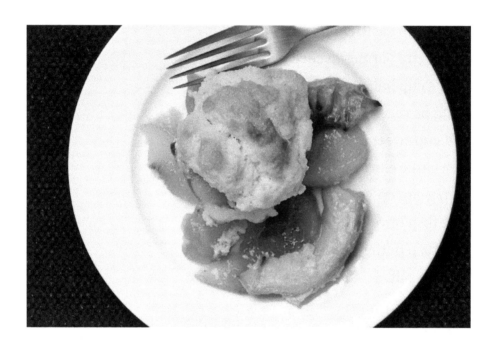

Tomato Corn Risotto

Preparation time: 10 minutes | Cooking Time: 13 minutes | Servings: 4

Ingredients:

1 1/2 cups arborio rice

1 cup cherry tomatoes, halved

1/4 cup basil, chopped

1/4 cup parmesan cheese, grated

1/4 cup half and half

32 oz vegetable broth

1 cup sweet corn

3 garlic cloves, minced

1/2 cup onion, chopped

2 tbsp olive oil

4 tbsp butter

1 tsp salt

Directions:

Add butter into the Pressure Pot and set the pot on sauté mode.

Add garlic and onion and sauté for 5 minutes.

Add rice and cook for 2-3 minutes.

Add broth, corn, pepper, and salt and stir well.

Seal pot with lid and cook on high pressure for 6 minutes.

Once done then release pressure using the quick-release method then open the lid.

Stir in cherry tomatoes, basil, parmesan, and a half and half.
Serve and enjoy.

Nutrition:

Calories 548, Fat 24g, Carbohydrates 69.6g, Sugar 3.8g, Protein 14.1g, Cholesterol 41mg.

Pancetta & Spinach Frittata

Preparation time: 15 minutes | Cooking Time: 16 minutes | Servings: 2

Ingredients:

¼ cup pancetta

½ of tomato, cubed

¼ cup fresh baby spinach

3 eggs

Salt and ground black pepper, as required

¼ cup parmesan cheese, grated

Directions:

Heat a nonstick skillet over medium heat and cook the pancetta for about 5 minutes.

Add the tomato and spinach cook for about 2-3 minutes.

Remove from the heat and drain the grease from the skillet.

Set aside to cool slightly.

Meanwhile, in a small bowl, add the eggs, salt, and black pepper and beat well.

In the bottom of a greased baking pan, place the pancetta mixture and top with the eggs, followed by the cheese.

Press the "power button" of the air fry oven and turn the dial to select the "air fry" mode.

Press the time button and again turn the dial to set the cooking time to 8 minutes.

Now push the temp button and rotate the dial to set the temperature at 355° F.

Press the "start/pause" button to start.

When the unit beeps to show that it is preheated, open the lid.

Arrange pan over the "wire rack" and insert in the oven.

Cut into equal-sized wedges and serve.

Nutrition:

Calories 28, Total fat 20.8g, Saturated fat 7.2g, Cholesterol 285mg, Sodium 915mg, Total carbs 1.7g, Fiber 0.3g, Sugar 0.9g, Protein 23.1 g.

Bacon, Mushroom & Tomato Frittata

Preparation time: 15 minutes | Cooking Time: 16 minutes | Servings: 2

Ingredients:

1 cooked bacon slice, chopped

6 cherry tomatoes, halved

6 fresh mushrooms, sliced

Salt and ground black pepper, as required

3 eggs

1 tablespoon fresh parsley, chopped

¼ cup parmesan cheese, grated

Directions:

In a baking pan, add the bacon, tomatoes, mushrooms, salt, and black pepper and mix well.

Press the "power button" of the air fry oven and turn the dial to select the "air fry" mode.

Press the time button and again turn the dial to set the cooking time to 16 minutes.

Now push the temp button and rotate the dial to set the temperature at 320° F.

Press the "start/pause" button to start.

When the unit beeps to show that it is preheated, open the lid.

Arrange pan over the "wire rack" and insert in the oven.

Meanwhile, in a bowl, add the eggs and beat well.

Add the parsley and cheese and mix well.

After 6 minutes of cooking, top the bacon mixture with egg mixture evenly.

Cut into equal-sized wedges and serve.

Nutrition:

Calories 228, Total fat 15.5g, Saturated fat 5.3g, Cholesterol 270mg, Sodium 608mg, Total carbs 3.5g, Fiber 0.9g, Sugar 2.1g, Protein 19.8g.

Veggie Pastry

Preparation Time: 30 minutes, | Cooking Time: 20 minutes | Servings: 4

Ingredients:

1 tbsp Chopped chives

½ cup Chopped kale

½ cup Chopped Bok Choy

½ cup Almond milk

Whisked eggs

1 tbsp Avocado oil

A pinch of salt and pepper

Directions:

Mix the chives, kale, Bok Choy, almond milk, eggs, salt, and pepper in a bowl.

Coat the muffin pastry tray with oil and pour the mix into it.

Pour the 1 and 1/2 cups of water into the Pressure Pot, put it in the inner pot, and place the pastry tray inside it. Seal the lid to cook for 20 minutes at high pressure.

Natural release the pressure for 10 minutes and let the pastry cool down and serve.

Nutrition:

Calories 142, fat 12g, carbs 3.3g, protein 6.7g, fiber 1.1g.

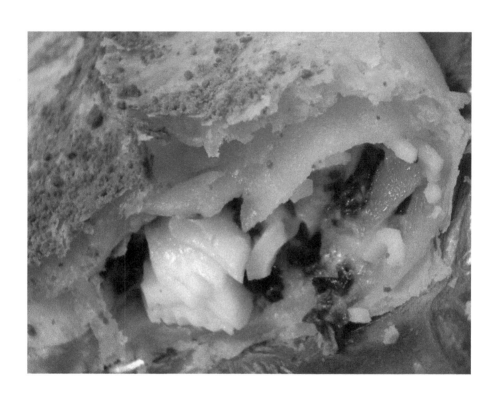

103

Artichoke and Spinach Scones

Preparation Time: 30 minutes, | Cooking Time: 20 minutes |
Servings: 12

Ingredients:

Eggs

1 cup Baby spinach; chopped

2 cup Canned artichoke hearts; drained and chopped

cups Almond flour

1 tsp Baking soda

A pinch of salt and black pepper

Cooking spray

Directions:

Combine the eggs, spinach, baking soda, artichoke hearts, almond flour, salt, and pepper in a bowl and set aside.

Coat the muffin tray with cooking spray and pour the spinach mix in the tray.

Pour the 1 ½ cups water into the Pressure Pot and place the inner pot inside it. Put the muffin tray inside the pot and seal the lid to cook for 20 minutes at high pressure.

Natural release the pressure for 10 minutes and let the scones cool and serve.

Nutrition:

Calories 66, fat 4.5g, carbs 0.6g, protein 5.8g, fiber 0.2g.

Nutty Coconut Mousse

Preparation Time: 10 minutes, | Cooking Time: 20 minutes |
Servings: 6

Ingredients:

2 cups Coconut milk

½ cup Unsweetened and shredded coconut

¼ cup Chopped walnuts

1 cup Coconut cream

Directions:

Mix all the ingredients in the Pressure Pot and seal the lid to
cook for 5 minutes at high pressure.

Quick-release the pressure for 5 minutes, share into bowls, and
serve.

Nutrition:

Calories 332, fat 33.8g, carbs 7.8g, protein 4.2g, fiber 3.6g.

Creamy Zucchini

Preparation Time: 22 minutes, | Cooking Time: 20 minutes |
Servings: 4

Ingredients:

Sliced zucchini

1 tbsp Chopped dill

½ cup Veggie stock

½ cup Softened cream cheese

½ cup Heavy cream

A pinch of salt and black pepper

1 tbsp Avocado oil

2 cloves minced garlic

Directions:

Put the zucchini in the Pressure Pot and mix in the stock, salt,
and pepper then seal the lid to cook for 12 minutes at high
pressure.

Natural release the pressure for 10 minutes, strain the zucchini,
and put it in a food processor. Mix in the rest of the ingredients
and blend well. Share into bowls and serve as a spread.

Nutrition:

Calories 193, fat 16.5g, carbs 7.8g, protein 5.2g, fiber 2.5g.

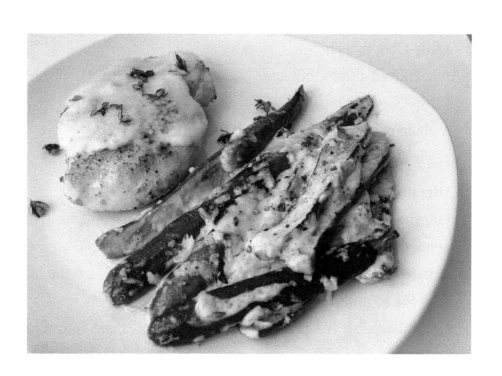

Cheesy Radish and Tomatoes Jumble

Preparation Time: 20 minutes, | Cooking Time: 20 minutes | Servings: 4

Ingredients:

¼ cup Sliced radishes

½ cup Shredded mozzarella

1 tbsp Chopped chives

1 lb. Halved cherry tomatoes

1 tbsp Chopped basil

A pinch of salt and black pepper

1 tbsp Olive oil

Directions:

Put the chives, radishes, basil, tomatoes, olive oil, salt, and pepper inside the Pressure Pot and mix it well.

Drizzle the mozzarella cheese over the spread and seal the lid to cook for 10 minutes at high pressure.

Natural release the pressure for 10 minutes, share into plates, and serve.

Nutrition:

Calories 62, fat 4.4g, carbs 4.9g, protein 2.1g, fiber 1.5g.

Garlic Pork Meat with Kale

Preparation Time: 25 minutes, | Cooking Time: 20 minutes | Servings: 4

Ingredients:

1 Lb. Torn kale

1 Chopped spring onion

½ cup Beef stock

2 cups Ground pork meat

A pinch of salt and black pepper

1 tbsp Avocado oil

2 cloves minced garlic

Directions:

Press 'Sauté' on the Pressure Pot and pour in the oil. When hot, add the garlic, onion, and pork meat to brown for 5 minutes.

Mix in the kale, spring onion, beef stock, salt, and pepper, and seal the lid to cook for 10 minutes on high pressure.

Natural release the pressure for 10 minutes, share into plates, and serve.

Nutrition:

Calories 66, fat 5.3g, carbs 6.5g, protein 3.8g, fiber 2g.

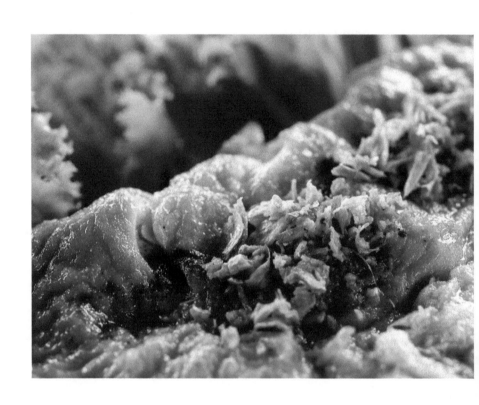

Lightning Source UK Ltd.
Milton Keynes UK
UKHW020817170621
385664UK00001B/105

9 781803 175232